Pediatric Allergies

A CLINICAL SUPPORT CHART

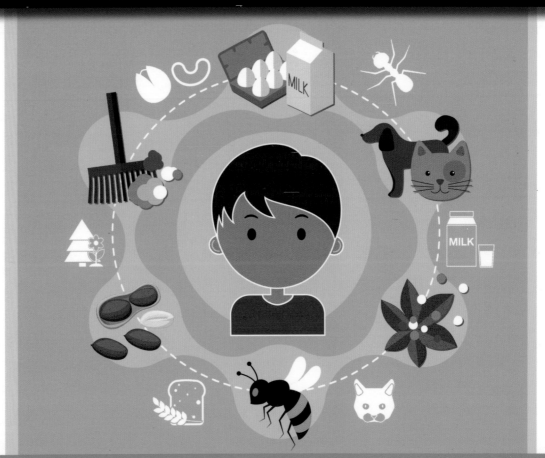

American Academy of Pediatrics

DEDICATED TO THE HEALTH OF ALL CHILDREN®

Contents

1 Tab 1
Allergic Conjunctivitis

2 Tab 2
Allergic Rhinitis

4 Tab 3
Respiratory Exposures

6 Tab 4
Remediation Strategies for Common Respiratory Allergens

8 Tab 5
Mold Exposures

10 Tab 6
Mold-Related Illness and Health Effects

12 Tab 7
Hymenoptera Venom Allergy

14 Tab 8
Classic Reactions to Antibiotics

16 Tab 9
Immediate Reactions to Antibiotics

18 Tab 10
Nonimmediate Reactions to Antibiotics

20 Tab 11
Nickel Allergy

22 Tab 12
Latex Allergy

24 Tab 13
Diagnosis of Atopic Dermatitis

26 Tab 14
Treatment of Atopic Dermatitis

28 Tab 15
Avoiding Eczema Triggers

30 Tab 16
Food Allergies

32 Tab 17
Cow's Milk Allergy

34 Tab 18
Peanut Allergy

36 Tab 19
Anaphylaxis Recognition

38 Tab 20
Anaphylaxis Treatment

42 Tab 21
AAP Allergy and Anaphylaxis Emergency Plan

44 Tab 22
Allergy testing

46 Tab 23
Immunotherapy

Pediatric Allergies: A Clinical Support Chart

Thank you to the American Academy of Pediatrics Section on Allergy and Immunology for their expert review.

American Academy of Pediatrics Publishing Staff
Mary Lou White, *Chief Product and Services Officer/SVP, Membership, Marketing, and Publishing*
Mark Grimes, *Vice President, Publishing*
Heather Babiar, MS, *Senior Editor, Professional/Clinical Publishing*
Theresa Wiener, *Production Manager, Clinical and Professional Publications*
Mary Louise Carr, MBA, *Marketing Manager, Clinical Publications*

Published by the American Academy of Pediatrics
345 Park Blvd
Itasca, IL 60143
Telephone: 630/626-6000
Facsimile: 847/434-8000
www.aap.org

The American Academy of Pediatrics is an organization of 67,000 primary care pediatricians, pediatric medical subspecialists, and pediatric surgical specialists dedicated to the health, safety, and well-being of all infants, children, adolescents, and young adults.

While every effort has been made to ensure the accuracy of this publication, the American Academy of Pediatrics does not guarantee that it is accurate, complete, or without error.

The recommendations in this publication do not indicate an exclusive course of treatment or serve as a standard of medical care. Variations, taking into account individual circumstances, may be appropriate.

Any websites, brand names, products, or manufacturers are mentioned for informational and identification purposes only and do not imply an endorsement by the American Academy of Pediatrics (AAP). The AAP is not responsible for the content of external resources. Information was current at the time of publication.

The publishers have made every effort to trace the copyright holders for borrowed materials. If they have inadvertently overlooked any, they will be pleased to make the necessary arrangements at the first opportunity.

This publication has been developed by the American Academy of Pediatrics. No commercial involvement of any kind has been solicited or accepted in the development of the content of this publication.

Every effort has been made to ensure that the drug selection and dosages set forth in this publication are in accordance with the current recommendations and practice at the time of publication. It is the responsibility of the health care professional to check the package insert of each drug for any change in indications or dosage and for added warnings and precautions.

Every effort is made to keep *Pediatric Allergies: A Clinical Support Chart* consistent with the most recent advice and information available from the American Academy of Pediatrics.

Please visit www.aap.org/errata for an up-to-date list of any applicable errata for this publication.

Special discounts are available for bulk purchases of this publication. Email Special Sales at nationalaccounts@aap.org for more information.

Printed in the United States of America
9-493/0323   1 2 3 4 5 6 7 8 9 10

MA1082
ISBN: 978-1-61002-663-5
eBook: 978-1-61002-664-2

Cover and publication design by LSD DESIGN LLC

The American Academy of Pediatrics is committed to principles of equity, diversity, and inclusion in its publishing program. Editorial boards, author selections, and author transitions (publication succession plans) are designed to include diverse voices that reflect society as a whole. Editor and author teams are encouraged to actively seek out diverse authors and reviewers at all stages of the editorial process. Publishing staff are committed to promoting equity, diversity, and inclusion in all aspects of publication writing, review, and production.

TAB 1

Allergic Conjunctivitis

Atopic allergic conjunctivitis is largely an immunoglobulin E-mediated reaction, often to airborne allergens. Treatment of allergic conjunctivitis should be based on the severity of symptoms and can include topical and systemic antihistamines, topical mast-cell stabilizers, topical nonsteroidal anti-inflammatory agents, and selective use of topical corticosteroids for severe cases. It is important to remember that other atopic conditions, such as allergic rhinitis and asthma, are often present and must also be treated.

Allergic Conjunctivitis

Cause	Allergens or irritants cause the protective outer covering of the eye to become swollen and inflamed.
Symptoms	■ Ocular pruritus, erythema, and clear/white discharge when exposed to sensitized aeroallergens ■ Burning ■ Swelling of the eyelid ■ Blurred vision ■ Sensitivity to light
Other features	■ May be acute or chronic ■ Almost always associated with itching ■ Discharge may be clear with some mucus, or stringy and white ■ Conjunctival edema with associated redness may appear as an intensely swollen eye
Environmental triggers	■ Pollen ■ Mold/fungi ■ Dust mites ■ Pet/animal dander ■ Cockroaches
Irritants	■ Cigarette smoke ■ Contact lenses ■ Contact lens solution ■ Cosmetics ■ Perfume
Treatment	■ Antihistamines ■ Eye drops ■ However, the most effective treatment for eye allergies is avoiding environmental triggers and irritants

Derived from Kneen L. Red eye/pinkeye. *Pediatric Care Online.* https://publications.aap.org/pediatriccare/article/doi/10.1542/aap.ppcqr.396107/1547/Red-Eye-Pink-Eye. Updated August 12, 2022. Accessed August 26, 2022; and All about allergies. Allergy and Asthma Network. https://allergyasthmanetwork.org/allergies. Accessed August 26, 2022.

Differentiating Types of Conjunctivitis

	Bacterial	Viral	Allergic	Probable Referral
Presentation	Unilateral or bilateral	Usually unilateral, then spreads to other eye	Usually bilateral: unusually can be unilateral with specific exposures	
Season	Common in winter	Spring or fall	Spring, summer and fall, or year-round indoor allergens can be triggers	
Onset	Concurrent with otitis media	Concurrent systemic viral infection	Acute or chronic	
Symptoms	Crusting on eyelashes Gluey or sticky eyelids ± fever	Tearing Eye irritation ± fever	Itching Conjunctival edema Swelling of eyelids	Light sensitivity Pain Blurred vision
Discharge type	Purulent, thick, yellow/green	Serous or mucoid	Stringy, whitish ropey, if any	
Patient type	Younger children Contact lens wearer	Any age	>2 years	Red eye/discharge for ≥2 weeks
Examination findings	Papules on conjunctiva	Follicles on palpebral conjunctiva Frequent preauricular nodes	Conjunctival edema and injection	Purulent discharge

From Kneen L. Red eye/pinkeye. *Pediatric Care Online.* https://publications.aap.org/pediatriccare/article/doi/10.1542/aap.ppcqr.396107/1547/Red-Eye-Pink-Eye. Updated August 12, 2022. Accessed August 26, 2022.

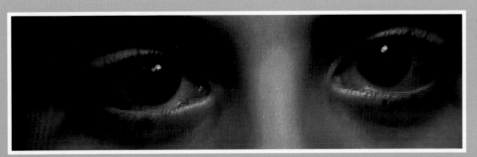

Allergic conjunctivitis. Note mild bilateral conjunctival injection and bilateral lower lid shines with dark lower lids.

From Wright KW, Strube YN. *Pediatric Ophthalmology.* 4th ed. American Academy of Pediatrics; 2019.

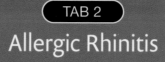

TAB 2

Allergic Rhinitis

Allergic Rhinitis Overview

Manifestation	Symptoms such as nasal congestion, rhinorrhea, sneezing, and itching
Symptoms	Can be variable, depending on: - Seasonal exposure to pollens from trees, grasses, molds, fungi, and weeds - Perennial symptoms, which can be triggered by allergens such as dust mites, molds, fungi, cockroaches, and pets
Diagnosis	Characterized by > 1 of the following nasal symptoms: congestion, rhinorrhea, postnasal drip, sneezing, and itching or allergic conjunctivitis symptoms, such as itchy, watery eyes. Two elements are often necessary to establish the diagnosis of allergic rhinitis: - Symptoms consistent with allergic rhinitis - Positive skin test results or serum IgE test results for seasonal and/or perennial aeroallergens, which need to correlate with the clinical history The diagnosis can also be assigned with a strong clinical history associated with known exposures, such as: - Worsening of symptoms around pets or other known triggers - Seasonal symptoms that correlate with a known regional pollen season
Causes	IgE-mediated hypersensitivity to aeroallergens, including pollens, dust mites, cockroaches, pets, molds, and fungi
How common?	One of the most common chronic illnesses in developed countries. Most commonly develops prior to the age of 20 but can manifest at any age.
Effects	Results in marked morbidity that includes decreased quality of life, missed school or workdays, and substantial treatment-related costs

Testing	Testing for allergic sensitizations may be performed with either of the following methods:
	- Skin prick testing
	  - Bioassay to evaluate the presence of allergen-specific IgE
	  - Involves scratching the skin with individual concentrated aeroallergens
	  - Results available within 15–20 minutes
	- Serum allergen-specific IgE testing
	  - Another option for assessing specific IgE to aeroallergens
	  - Sometimes less sensitive than skin testing for aeroallergens

Treatment strategies	- Oral H_1 antihistamines
	- Nasal steroids (in many patients, nasal steroids can also improve ocular symptoms)
	- Decongestants
	- Leukotriene blockers
	- Topical (eye drops) antihistamines and/or mast-cell stabilizers
	  - Olopatadine, bepotastine, azelastine, epinastine (prescription only)
	  - Cromolyn sodium
	  - Ketotifen
	- Immunotherapy

IgE, immunoglobulin E.

Derived from American Academy of Pediatrics Section on Pediatric Pulmonology and Sleep Medicine. *Pediatric Pulmonology, Asthma, and Sleep Medicine: A Quick Reference Guide*. Stokes DC, Dozor AJ, eds. American Academy of Pediatrics; 2018.

TAB 2

Allergic Rhinitis

Differentiating Factors for Common Causes of Rhinitis in Children

	Allergic Rhinitis	Nonallergic Rhinitis	Anatomic Abnormalities	Recurrent Viral Upper Respiratory Infections
Age of onset	≥ 12 mo for perennial 2–3 y for seasonal	≥3 mo	Can be present from birth	≥3 mo
Itching	Mild to severe itching	No itching	No itching	No itching
Mucus	Always clear or white	Clear	Clear	Clear or yellow/green
Congestion	Some congestion	Severe congestion	Some congestion	Some congestion
Fever	Never	No fever	No fever	Can occur with or without fever
Duration	Weeks to months	Months	Months	10–14 d

Derived from American Academy of Pediatrics Section on Pediatric Pulmonology and Sleep Medicine. *Pediatric Pulmonology, Asthma, and Sleep Medicine: A Quick Reference Guide.* Stokes DC, Dozor AJ, eds. American Academy of Pediatrics; 2018.

Common Medications Used to Treat Allergic Rhinitis

Drug Type	Common Examples	Discussion
Antihistamines		
First-generation H₁ antihistamines	Diphenhydramine, chlorpheniramine	▪ Effective agents for rhinitis symptoms but often limited by side effect profiles ▪ Side effects can include sedation, dry eyes, dry mouth
Second-generation H₁ antihistamines	Loratadine, fexofenadine, cetirizine	▪ First-line therapy for rhinitis ▪ Inexpensive and safe ▪ Safe for long-term use, given the side effect profile
Intranasal antihistamines	Azelastine, olopatadine	Used as an add-on therapy in allergic rhinitis and often effective in other types of rhinitis, such as nonallergic rhinitis
Topical Corticosteroids		
Topical (intranasal) corticosteroids	Beclomethasone, budesonide, ciclesonide, flunisolide, fluticasone furoate, fluticasone propionate, mometasone, triamcinolone	▪ Intranasal corticosteroids are an effective medication class for controlling symptoms of allergic rhinitis. ▪ The regular use of intranasal corticosteroids is generally preferred over as-needed use. ▪ Fluticasone furoate, mometosone, and triamcinolone are approved for use in patients as young as 2 y of age.
Leukotriene Blockers		
LTRAs, 5-LO inhibitors	LTRAs: montelukast, zafirlukast 5-LO inhibitor: zileuton	▪ Not a first-line treatment for rhinitis but can have a role as an add-on therapy ▪ Can improve rhinorrhea, sneezing, and pruritus in patients with allergic rhinitis ▪ Often used if there is concomitant asthma ▪ LTRAs are generally preferred over 5-LO inhibitors, given that liver function needs to be monitored with 5-LO inhibitors. ▪ Montelukast is approved in patients as young as 6 mo of age. ▪ Zafirlukast is approved in patients ≥5 y of age. ▪ Zileuton is approved in patients ≥12 y of age.
Decongestants		
	Oxymetazoline, phenylephrine, pseudoephedrine	▪ While these agents work well for short-term relief of congestion, they should not be used long-term, given the side effect profile. ▪ Medications such as oxymetazoline are approved in children ≥6 y of age.

LTRA, leukotriene receptor antagonist; 5-LO, 5-lipoxygenase.

From American Academy of Pediatrics Section on Pediatric Pulmonology and Sleep Medicine. *Pediatric Pulmonology, Asthma, and Sleep Medicine: A Quick Reference Guide.* Stokes DC, Dozor AJ, eds. American Academy of Pediatrics; 2018.

TAB 3

Respiratory Exposures

Respiratory irritants, toxins, and allergens can all contribute to a child's breathing problems. Problems can arise from indoor **and outdoor** sources; however, indoor exposures contribute most to respiratory symptoms in children. Exposure can occur in **the home**, at school, at day care, at play, or at work.

Note: The most important part of identifying an environmental contribution to a child's respiratory illness is the history of **relevant** exposures. The patient or parent may not connect the relevant exposure to the respiratory symptom. Often it is not **exclusively** one exposure that contributes to the respiratory symptoms but a combination of several.

Environmental Exposures and Sequelae

Irritants	Stimulate airway inflammation by a mechanism of action not dependent on prior sensitization
Toxins	Directly cause damage to airway or lung tissues

Common indoor respiratory irritants and toxins	■ Smoke from any source
	  – Common sources of smoke include tobacco, other substances of abuse, incense, fireplaces, wood-burning stoves, gas stoves, gas heaters, and kerosene heaters.
	  – Sometimes the source of smoke may be from a friend or neighbor. Smoking in multiunit housing involuntarily introduces smoke exposure to those who live in proximity to smokers.
	  – Although not technically smoke from combustion, the emissions from electronic nicotine delivery systems (ENDS) contain chemicals that are known respiratory irritants and toxins.
	■ Strong chemicals
	  – These include air fresheners, cleaning agents, and insecticides.
	  – Chemicals used in hobbies or home remodeling can be irritants or a source of toxic exposure.
	  – Ask about exposure to formaldehyde due to off-gassing from building materials, household products (glues, paints, finishes, etc), and products of combustion (from gas stoves, kerosene space heaters, tobacco smoke, etc).

Allergens	■ Airway inflammation is stimulated by an allergic mechanism. ■ Mast cells, eosinophils, and immunoglobulin E play important roles in allergic reactions. ■ The individual needs to have been previously sensitized (ie, allergic) for exposure to the allergen to be a problem. Seasonal allergies are uncommon prior to the second year after birth. ■ Relevant allergens are usually inhaled. It is unusual for a food allergy to cause only respiratory symptoms.
Common indoor respiratory allergens	■ Dust mites ■ House pets ■ Rodent infestation ■ Cockroach secretions and droppings ■ Mold and mildew
Common outdoor respiratory allergens	■ Pollens of trees, grasses, and weeds ■ Mold
Hypersensitivity pneumonitis	■ Organic and inorganic antigens can trigger a T-cell–mediated reaction in sensitized persons. ■ Acute and subacute hypersensitivity pneumonitis can mimic pneumonia. ■ Chronic hypersensitivity pneumonitis can lead to pulmonary fibrosis and severe lung disease. ■ Implicated antigens include avian (bird) antigens, fungi and fungal spores, bacterial antigens, and low-molecular- weight chemicals. ■ This type of reaction is uncommon; however, it is important to recognize.

TAB 3

Respiratory Exposures

When to Refer

Refer the patient to a board-certified allergist	<ul><li>If symptoms are uncontrolled despite first-line therapies, such as antihistamines, intranasal corticosteroids, antileukotrienes, leukotriene antagonists, and nasal antihistamines</li><li>When patients or parents want to try and limit medication use by avoiding specific allergens</li><li>When patients are using decongestants inappropriately</li><li>If skin testing is needed to identify sensitization to inhalant allergens</li><li>If immunotherapy is being considered</li></ul>
Refer the family for a home environmental assessment	<ul><li>If an environmental trigger is suspected for a severe lung disease but not identifiable from the history alone</li><li>For additional help with identifying and reducing exposure to relevant environmental triggers</li><li>If the local health department or the child's managed care program care manager may be able to arrange for the home assessment, especially if the child has severe lung disease. Quality of services, if available, can vary. Pediatricians should be aware of available resources in their community. To avoid adverse incentives, it is prudent to not have the same companies perform both assessment and remediation.</li><li>If a home assessment visit cannot be accomplished, asking for pictures of the home (indoor and outdoor) may help to identify potential environmental triggers.</li><li>Refer the family to social services or relevant community resources if needed to address problems with housing quality or homelessness.</li></ul>

Adapted from American Academy of Pediatrics Section on Pediatric Pulmonology and Sleep Medicine. *Pediatric Pulmonology, Asthma, and Sleep Medicine: A Quick Reference Guide.* Stokes DC, Dozor AJ, eds. American Academy of Pediatrics; 2018.

TAB 4

Remediation Strategies for Common Respiratory Allergens

Pollen	Pollens of trees, grasses, and weeds can contribute to allergic respiratory symptoms.

Remediation strategies	▪ Before going out, check the daily pollen count in your area at www.airnow.gov.
	▪ Know the pollen seasons in your area. In most areas:
	  – *Tree* pollen levels are highest in the late winter to early spring.
	  – *Grass* pollen levels are highest in the spring to summer.
	  – *Weed* pollen levels are highest in the late summer to fall.
	▪ Stay inside and keep windows closed when pollen levels are high—usually in the morning to midafternoon.
	▪ Remember to use any necessary respiratory medications before going out.
	▪ For individuals with specific allergies, immunotherapy may provide substantial relief from allergic symptoms.

Dust mites	House dust mites thrive on humidity and shed skin, both of which are in ample supply in beds and bedding. Dust mites also thrive in the fabric of carpets and upholstered furniture. Dust mites do not grow well in areas of low humidity (< 40%).
Remediation strategies	▪ Encase the child's mattress, box spring, and pillow in allergen-proof covers. ▪ Wash bedding in hot water weekly (130° F). Wash curtains often. ▪ Minimize the number of stuffed animals on the child's bed, and wash them weekly in hot water. Alternatively, after an initial washing, they can be run through a dryer on high heat once a week. ▪ Use a dehumidifier to reduce indoor humidity to < 40% (may not be possible in very humid areas). ▪ Air filters are not helpful for dust mite allergens, as they fall out of the air quickly. ▪ Vacuum twice per week, and use a vacuum cleaner with a HEPA filter. Dust the home frequently.
Animals/pets	Allergens including the dander (shed skin), saliva, and urine of furry or feathered pets may stay airborne for long periods.
Remediation strategies	▪ The best approach is to remove the pet from the home or keep the pet outside only. It may take months for allergen levels to decrease after a pet is removed. ▪ If removal of the pet is not an option, keep the pet out of the child's bedroom, bathe the pet weekly, and use HEPA filters, especially in the child's bedroom. ▪ Balance the importance of the pet to the family against the severity of allergic symptoms. It is not necessary to advise removing pets from the home unless specific allergic sensitization is documented.
Rodents	Rodent infestation can be an important allergy and asthma trigger.
Remediation strategies	▪ Find and close holes in walls and around plumbing. ▪ Do not leave food or water out. ▪ If using rodent poisons, keep them well out of reach of children. ▪ Consider calling an integrated pest management professional.

TAB 5

Mold Exposures

Recommendations to Pediatricians

1 Because there are established health hazards, inquire about the presence of mold as part of a "healthy-home" inventory. Questions about a child's environment are basic to a comprehensive pediatric health history. Questions can be incorporated during visits for health supervision or sick visits. Asking about a child's environment should be routine for children with common illnesses, such as allergic rhinitis/conjunctivitis and asthma, as well as for those with less common illnesses, such as hypersensitivity pneumonitis.

2 Provide guidance to parents of all children about

   a. the adverse health effects of mold exposure, especially the causal relationship between mold and allergic illness and respiratory symptoms, and

   b. preventing and reducing mold exposure in the immediate indoor and outdoor environments.

3 Educate families on mold remediation. Visible signs of mold growth (eg, discolored patches or cottony or speckled growth on walls or furniture, evidence of dampness or water damage inside the home, or an earthy musty odor in a particular area) suggest a damp environment and mold growth. In areas where flooding has occurred, prompt cleaning (within 24 hours) of walls and other flood-damaged items is necessary to prevent mold growth. Testing the environment for specific molds is usually not necessary. In general, individuals can perform mold cleanup for areas less than 10 feet.

4 When treating an infant with AIPH, inquire about mold and water damage in the home. Report cases of AIPH to state health departments. Avoidance of exposure to mold and secondhand cigarette smoke is always recommended, but especially in cases of AIPH.

5 Be aware that there are no uniformly accepted, valid, quantitative environmental sampling methods or serologic tests to assess exposure to mold and other agents associated with damp indoor environments. There are also no accepted valid airborne levels of mold that predict adverse health effects.

6 Be aware that there is currently no method to test humans for toxigenic mold exposure.

7 Be aware that mold-contaminated foods (especially grains) can contain harmful amounts of mycotoxins. The US Department of Agriculture has set allowable limits in certain food items and has some routine monitoring in place to prevent harmful ingestion of mycotoxin-contaminated foods. Inquire about dietary history if a mycotoxin-induced illness is suspected.

AIPH, Acute idiopathic pulmonary hemorrhage. Adapted from American Academy of Pediatrics Committee on Environmental Health. Spectrum of noninfectious health effects from molds. *Pediatrics.* 2006;118(6):2582–2586.

TAB 6

Mold-Related Illness and Health Effects

Guidelines for Pediatricians Considering Possible Illness Related to Damp, Moldy Indoor Spaces

When to consider indoor mold-related illness[a]
- Chronic respiratory symptoms of unclear etiology
- Poorly controlled asthma, perennial allergic rhinitis, or chronic sinusitis
- Respiratory symptoms or recurrent influenza-like symptoms in a moldy environment
- Suspected or diagnosed hypersensitivity pneumonitis, allergic bronchopulmonary aspergillosis, or fungal sinusitis
- Unexplained pulmonary hemorrhage, especially in infants

Assessing exposure to mold: helpful questions
- Have you seen any mold or mildew on walls, floors, ceilings, or carpets, including your basement (discolored patches or cottony or speckled growth on walls or furniture)?
- Have you noticed a musty or earthy smell indoors?
- Has the home been flooded?
- Does the home contain any water-damaged wood or cardboard?
- Has there been a roof or plumbing leak, standing water in the home, or areas with chronic dampness/moisture, including the basement?
- Is there often condensation (fog) on the inside of the windows and/or cold inside surfaces?
- Have humidifiers or air-conditioner drip pans been checked for mold overgrowth?
- Are symptoms better away from the house?
- Describe the conditions of your basement, dwellings, and school or other places where you routinely spend time.

Environmental assessment
- Work with an experienced industrial hygienist or investigator.
- Methods: visual inspection, bulk sampling, and air sampling of visible or culturable fungal spores
- Serologic testing of allergen-specific immunoglobulin E may be helpful.[a]

[a] Physicians should also consider and rule out other possible non–mold-related etiologies.

From Mazur LJ, Kim J; American Academy of Pediatrics Committee on Environmental Health. Spectrum of noninfectious health effects from molds. *Pediatrics.* 2006;118(6):e1909–e1926.

TAB 6

Mold-Related Illness and Health Effects

Mycotoxin-Producing Molds and Their Health Effects

Fungus	Mycotoxin	Adverse Health Effect
Alternaria alternate	Tenuazonic acid	Hepatotoxic, nephrotoxic, hemorrhagic
Aspergillus flavus	Aflatoxins	Hepatotoxic, carcinogenic
Aspergillus fumigatus	Fumitremorgens	Tremorgenic
Aspergillus nidulans	Sterigmatocystin	Hepatotoxic, carcinogenic
Aspergillus ochraceus	Ochratoxin A	Hepatotoxic, nephrotoxic, carcinogenic
Cladosporium species	Epicladosporic acid	
Fusarium moniliforme	Fumonisins	Neurotoxic, hepatotoxic, nephrotoxic
Fusarium poae	T-2 toxin	Hemorrhagic, immunosuppressive
Fusarium sporotrichioides	Trichothecenes	Causes alimentary tract aleukia (nausea, vomiting)
Penicillium expansum	Patulin	Nephrotoxic, carcinogenic
	Citrinin	
Penicillium griseofulvum	Griseofulvin	Hepatotoxic, carcinogenic, teratogenic
Pithomyces chartarum	Sporidesmin	Hepatotoxic; causes photosensitization, eczema
	Phylloerythrin	
Stachybotrys chartarum	Satratoxins	Immunosuppressive, hematotoxic
	Verrucarins	Inflammatory, immunosuppressive
	Roridins	Causes dermatitis; hematotoxic, hemorrhagic

From Mazur LJ, Kim J; American Academy of Pediatrics Committee on Environmental Health. Spectrum of noninfectious health effects from molds. *Pediatrics.* 2006;118(6):e1909–e1926.

TAB 7

Hymenoptera Venom Allergy

Sources of Hymenoptera Venom

Most allergic reactions triggered by insect venom are from insects in the order Hymenoptera, especially the following:

- Yellow jackets
- Hornets
- Wasps (especially paper wasps)
- Bees
- Red ants ("fire ants")

Systemic Allergic Reactions

- Life-threatening systemic reactions secondary to insect stings occur in approximately 0.4%–0.8% of the pediatric population.
- Systemic reactions may present with variable symptoms ranging from mild to severe, with anaphylaxis (see Tab 19), including hypotension or the involvement of at least 2 organ systems.
- Symptoms of severe reactions can include:
  - Shortness of breath
  - Wheezing
  - Coughing
  - Pallor
  - Weak pulse
  - Fainting
  - Tight throat
  - Trouble breathing
  - Swelling of the lips or tongue that affects breathing
  - Hives
  - Confusion
- Given the high frequency of asymptomatic sensitization, venom testing should not be used for screening purposes.
- Children with symptoms limited to the skin (eg, local swelling, flushing, pruritus, and urticaria) are considered to have low risk for a more severe reaction.

Allergy Testing for Venom

- For children with large local reactions, there is <10% chance of a systemic reaction (usually milder than the index event) and <5% chance of anaphylaxis. Thus, venom testing is not indicated in children with isolated cutaneous symptoms.
- A patient who has experienced a life-threatening systemic reaction after an insect sting or bite should have testing performed by an allergist because the risk of anaphylaxis with subsequent stings is 30%–40% in children.
- Systemic anaphylaxis in any age group and generalized urticaria in adolescents older than 16 years warrant testing.
- Skin prick testing and intradermal testing are considered the standard means of diagnosis for venom allergy. However, serum immunoglobulin E tests for venom or venom components should be performed when skin test results are negative and the patient's history is suggestive of allergy to venom because a positive serum test result along with a negative skin test result indicates a risk for a systemic reaction.
- Serum tryptase should be tested in children with severe anaphylactic reactions.

Immunotherapy

- When anaphylactic allergy to venom is confirmed via skin testing, immunotherapy is indicated and can be highly effective (see Tab 23).
- Immunotherapy to identified insects can dramatically reduce the risk of future systemic reactions.

Toxic Reactions

- Insect stings can also cause serious symptoms that are *not* allergic. A toxic reaction occurs when the insect venom acts like a poison and causes symptoms similar to those of an allergic reaction, including:
  - Rapid swelling at the sting site
  - Headache
  - Weakness
  - Lightheadedness
  - Drowsiness
  - Fever
  - Diarrhea
  - Muscle spasms
  - Fainting (syncope)
  - Shock
  - Seizures
  - Death
- A toxic reaction can occur after only one sting, but it usually takes many stings from insects.
- Results of allergy testing are negative in this case.

When to Refer

- Refer patients to an allergist if they develop severe allergic reactions to insect bites, especially repeatedly, or if Hymenoptera allergy is suspected.
- Refer patients to an allergist if they should undergo allergy testing and/or immunotherapy or other dedicated treatment for apparent Hymenoptera venom allergy.

When to Admit

- Admit if the patient has a severe systemic allergic reaction, such as anaphylaxis, to an insect bite or sting.
- Admit if the patient needs intravenous antibiotics to treat secondary bacterial infection, cellulitis, or systemic infection from a sting or bite.
- Admit if the patient develops acute noninfectious complications, such as acute postinfectious glomerulonephritis and hypertension.
- Admit if the patient is suspected of having contracted viral meningitis or other severe or systemic illness through insect bites.

Derived from Wong AG, Lomas JM. Allergy testing and immunotherapy. *Pediatr Rev.* 2019;40(5):219–228; Sicherer SH, Wood RA; American Academy of Pediatrics Section on Allergy and Immunology. Allergy testing in childhood: using allergen-specific IgE tests. *Pediatrics.* 2012;129(1):193–197; and Stein DH, Barnett NK. Insect bites and infestations. In: McInerny TK, Adam HM, Campbell DE, et al, eds. *American Academy of Pediatrics Textbook of Pediatric Care.* 2nd ed. American Academy of Pediatrics; 2020. https://publications.aap.org/pediatriccare/book/348/chapter/5782048/Insect-Bites-and-Infestations. Accessed August 26, 2022.

TAB 19

Anaphylaxis Recognition

Differential Diagnosis of Anaphylaxis

Diagnosis	Clinical Features
Angioedema	Swelling of the face, neck, and extremities without pruritus No acute respiratory or cardiovascular symptoms
Asthma	Patient may have had previous similar episodes No acute dermatologic, GI, or cardiovascular symptoms
Cardiac tamponade	Muffled heart sounds and presence of pericardial friction rub No acute dermatologic or GI symptoms
Cholinergic urticaria	Urticaria and wheezing occurring within 30 minutes of vigorous exercise
Croup	Barking cough, stridor, fever No acute dermatologic, GI, or cardiovascular symptoms
Food poisoning and scombroid poisoning	Vomiting, diarrhea, possible flushing No acute dermatologic, respiratory, or cardiovascular symptoms
Mastocytosis	Most often involves the skin Patient may have bone marrow and solid-organ infiltration Increased tryptase levels
Neuroendocrine tumor	Predominantly GI symptoms with intermittent flushing Increased catecholamine levels, vasoactive intestinal polypeptide levels, and neurokinin levels
Panic attack	Feeling of impending doom No acute dermatologic symptoms
Vancomycin infusion reaction	Infusion with vancomycin may mimic anaphylaxis Slowing the rate of infusion decreases symptoms
Urticaria	No acute GI, respiratory, or cardiovascular symptoms

GI, gastrointestinal.

From American Academy of Pediatrics Section on Hospital Medicine. *Caring for the Hospitalized Child: A Handbook of Inpatient Pediatrics.* Gershel JC, Rauch DA, eds. 3rd ed. American Academy of Pediatrics. Forthcoming 2023.

Additional Signs and Symptoms of Anaphylaxis

▶ Morbilliform rash

▶ Conjunctival erythema

▶ Pruritus and tightness in the throat

▶ Dysphagia

▶ Dysphonia

▶ Hoarseness

▶ Dry staccato cough

▶ Sensation of pruritus in the external auditory canals

▶ Nasal pruritus

▶ Nasal congestion

▶ Rhinorrhea

▶ Sneezing

▶ Chest pain

▶ Dysrhythmia

▶ Near-syncope

▶ Pallor

▶ Cyanosis

▶ Confusion/altered mental status

▶ Aura of doom

▶ Uterine contractions

▶ Sudden isolated hypotension without a known allergen exposure

TAB 20

Anaphylaxis Treatment

American Academy of Pediatrics: Summary of Epinephrine Use for Anaphylaxis

Epinephrine is the medication of choice for the initial treatment of anaphylaxis. If injected promptly, it is nearly always effective. Delayed injection can be associated with poor outcomes, including fatality. All other medications, including H_1 antihistamines and bronchodilators such as albuterol, provide adjunctive treatment but do not replace epinephrine. After treatment with epinephrine for anaphylaxis in community settings, it is important for patients to be assessed in an emergency department to determine whether additional interventions—including oxygen, intravenous fluids, and adjunctive medications—are needed.

When anaphylaxis occurs in health care settings, epinephrine (0.01 mg/kg [maximum dose: 0.3 mg in a prepubertal child and up to 0.5 mg in a teenager]) administered via intramuscular (IM) injection in the mid-outer thigh (vastus lateralis muscle) is recommended. IM epinephrine achieves peak epinephrine concentrations promptly and is safer than an intravenous bolus injection.

When anaphylaxis occurs in community settings, epinephrine autoinjectors (EAs) are preferred because of their ease of use and accuracy of dosing as compared with the use of an ampoule, syringe, and needle by laypersons or the use of an unsealed syringe prefilled with epinephrine. In the United States and Canada, EAs are currently available in 3 fixed doses: 0.10 mg, 0.15 mg, and 0.3 mg. International guidelines suggest that when using EAs, patients weighing 7.5–15 kg (16.5–33 lb) should receive the 0.1-mg dose; patients 15–25 kg (33–55 lb) should receive the 0.15-mg dose; and those weighing 25 kg (55 lb) or more should receive the 0.3-mg dose. If the 0.10-mg dose is not available, the 0.15-mg dose is a reasonable alternative.

Adapted from Sicherer SH, Simons FER; American Academy of Pediatrics Section on Allergy and Immunology. Epinephrine for first-aid management of anaphylaxis. *Pediatrics*. 2017;139(3):e20164006.

(TAB 21)

AAP Allergy and Anaphylaxis Emergency Plan

Allergy and Anaphylaxis Emergency Plan

American Academy of Pediatrics
DEDICATED TO THE HEALTH OF ALL CHILDREN®

Child's name: _____ **Date of plan:** _____

Additional Instructions:

Contacts

Call 911 / Rescue squad: _____

Doctor: _____ Phone: _____

Parent/Guardian: _____ Phone: _____

Parent/Guardian: _____ Phone: _____

Other Emergency Contacts

Name/Relationship: _____ Phone: _____

Name/Relationship: _____ Phone: _____

© 2017 American Academy of Pediatrics, Updated 03/2019. All rights reserved. Your child's doctor will tell you to do what's best for your child. This information should not take the place of talking with your child's doctor. Page 2 of 2.

Indications for Testing

- Allergy testing should generally only be performed if the results will affect management. If a diagnosis is strongly suspected, confirmatory testing may also be important to enable appropriate counseling and treatment.
- A thorough clinical history is just as, if not more, important than testing. Positive findings from skin prick testing (SPT), intradermal testing (IDT), or serum-specific immunoglobulin E (IgE) testing indicate only the presence of allergen-specific IgE, and these results alone are not enough to diagnose clinical allergy.
- SPT and serum test results may be either false positive or false negative. Therefore, a positive allergy test result represents sensitization only and not clinical allergy. Based on the combination of a suggestive history and (positive) testing results, it is the provider's responsibility to determine whether clinical allergy is present.
- Long-term symptoms of allergic rhinitis or conjunctivitis, recurrent sinusitis (especially seasonal), or concern for allergic asthma are indications for environmental allergen testing when symptoms are persistent, refractory to standard care, or could be improved by proper allergen avoidance or when patients and families are curious about identifying potential triggers.
- Skin testing is indicated when an anaphylactic reaction has occurred or symptoms suspicious of an IgE-mediated allergy (eg, hives, intractable vomiting) are demonstrated with ingestion of a specific food. Testing should occur 4–6 weeks after the reaction has occurred. Negative SPT results can be particularly helpful because the tests are highly sensitive, with a negative predictive accuracy of 85%–95%.
- Skin testing for penicillin allergy is well validated and reliable. Investigation of penicillin allergy should be performed for any patient with a history of cutaneous reaction to aminopenicillins. For medication classes other than penicillin, skin testing is performed with less frequency.
- Patients with moderate to severe uncontrolled atopic dermatitis despite optimal skin care may also benefit from allergy testing (to both environmental and food allergens) to identify potential triggers.

Skin Prick Testing

- SPT is the most common method of testing used by allergists and is typically preferred as an initial approach. When deemed appropriate, it can be performed in patients as young as 1 month of age. Although infants typically exhibit appropriate cutaneous reactivity to antigen, the wheal size produced by SPT can be smaller in this population than in older (preschool-aged) children to adults. Antigen is available commercially in an aqueous form or is created from fresh foods or medications.
- The specificity of SPT is 70%–95% for inhalant allergens and 30%–70% for food allergens. The sensitivity is 80%–90% for inhalant allergens and 20%–60% for food allergens, and it increases to as high as 90% when fresh foods are used.

Intradermal Testing

- With IDT, allergen extract is injected intracutaneously. As with SPT, the wheal and erythema that develop are measured and compared with positive and negative controls.
- This test should be performed only if the SPT results were negative because IDT is more sensitive but less specific. The risk of a systemic reaction to IDT is higher than with SPT.
- Intradermal testing is performed for aeroallergen, drug, and insect allergy but not food allergy, for safety reasons.

Serum Testing

- Serum testing is favored in certain situations, such as for patients who have diffuse skin disease or who are unable to discontinue the use of suppressive medications before testing. Serum-specific IgE testing is often used in conjunction with SPT to monitor the severity of food allergies and to further determine whether an oral food challenge may be indicated.
- Serum-specific IgE testing can be used to detect serum IgE antibodies for specific allergens. The average sensitivity compared with SPT has been reported to be approximately 70%–75%; thus, SPT is preferred.

Contraindications to Testing

- Contraindications to allergy skin testing include:
  - Uncontrolled asthma
  - Diffuse skin rash
  - Inability to discontinue antihistaminic medication for at least 3–7 days
  - Pregnancy
  - Generalized edema
- Concurrent use of β-blockers is also a relative contraindication because the symptoms of anaphylaxis may be amplified, and the response to epinephrine may be blunted.

Derived from Wong AG, Lomas JM. Allergy testing and immunotherapy. *Pediatr Rev.* 2019;40(5):219–228.

Benefits of Immunotherapy

- In cases of allergic rhinitis, immunotherapy can decrease nasal and ocular symptoms, as well as medication requirements.
- In cases of allergic asthma, therapy leads to a clinically significant reduction in asthma symptoms and medication use.
- Immunotherapy in children with allergic rhinitis can help prevent the subsequent development of allergic asthma.
- The clinical benefits of immunotherapy often persist after immunotherapy is discontinued.
- Although immunotherapy is a time commitment for the patient and the caretaker, the alternative is pharmacotherapy for symptomatic relief that would be continued indefinitely.

Indications

- Based on practice guidelines, allergy immunotherapy is indicated for the treatment of patients with allergic rhinitis, allergic conjunctivitis, allergic asthma, or stinging insect hypersensitivity who demonstrate evidence of specific immunoglobulin E (IgE) antibodies with a relevant history and positive allergy test results.
- According to the Expert Panel, subcutaneous immunotherapy is recommended for those who have allergic asthma and whose symptoms worsen after exposure to certain allergens.
- According to the Expert Panel, sublingual immunotherapy is not recommended.
- Immunotherapy has been shown to be effective in both allergic rhinitis and allergic asthma.
- Allergen immunotherapy has been shown to alter the underlying immune response to aeroallergens.
- Immunotherapy is often indicated in the following patients:
  - Patients with symptoms that are uncontrolled despite medical therapy and environmental controls
  - Those who do not tolerate medications or who would like to try to decrease medication use
  - Those with a documented IgE-mediated hypersensitivity that correlates with the clinical history
- Age indications: While there is no age cutoff, it is recommended that children should be old enough to understand why they are receiving the injection and are willing participants, given the number of injections needed over the course of a 3–5-year treatment period.

Mechanism of Action

Prolonged administration of immunotherapy has been associated with:
- Induction of regulatory T cells, resulting in suppression of the pro-inflammatory T helper (Th_2 and Th_1) cells
- Decreased allergen-specific lymphocyte proliferation
- Decreased specific immunoglobulin E (IgE) and increased specific immunoglobulin G4 response to aeroallergens

Prescribing Immunotherapy

- Clinicians prescribing immunotherapy should have knowledge of the aeroallergens prevalent locally, cross-reactivity between aeroallergens, the potential for allergen degradation caused by proteolytic enzymes within aeroallergens, initial dosing and subsequent titration schedules (see the sample regimen on this Tab), and patient-specific history and IgE sensitivities.
- While most immunotherapy is administered in allergy and immunology offices, personnel in a primary care office who are properly trained in administering immunotherapy and treating anaphylaxis can administer this therapy once prescribed by a specialist. This can improve patient access to care.
- Clinical evaluation of the patient every 6–12 months is recommended to assess effectiveness and tolerance. Duration is tailored to the individual patient, with lack of clinical effect and intolerable adverse effects being the most significant reasons to discontinue therapy.

Risks of Immunotherapy

- Most patients experience local reactions at the site of the immunotherapy injection (eg, local erythema, pruritis, swelling, pain).
- While the risk is very low, systemic reactions (anaphylaxis) can occur. Patients need to remain in the clinic for ≥30 minutes after injections to monitor them for anaphylaxis.
- Any clinic that administers appropriate doses of subcutaneous immunotherapy should have experience in the diagnosis and treatment of anaphylaxis and have access to advanced cardiovascular life support.
- Premedication with an oral antihistamine is advised before each injection to mitigate adverse reactions.
- Contraindications include uncontrolled asthma, the inability to communicate clearly to the physician should a reaction occur, concurrent use of β-blockers, and other comorbidities that weaken a patient's ability to survive a systemic allergic reaction. For venom immunotherapy in particular, the concurrent use of angiotensin converting enzyme inhibitors leads to a greater risk of more serious anaphylaxis to a sting.

Derived from American Academy of Pediatrics Section on Pediatric Pulmonology and Sleep Medicine. *Pediatric Pulmonology, Asthma, and Sleep Medicine: A Quick Reference Guide.* Stokes DC, Dozor AJ, eds. American Academy of Pediatrics; 2018; US Department of Health and Human Services, National Institutes of Health, and the National Heart, Lung, and Blood Institute. *2020 Focused Updates to the Asthma Management Guidelines: A Report From the National Asthma Education and Prevention Program Coordinating Committee Expert Panel Working Group.* 2020. https://www.nhlbi.nih.gov/health-topics/all-publications-and-resources/2020-focused-updates-asthma-management-guidelines. Accessed August 26, 2022; and Wong AG, Lomas JM. Allergy testing and immunotherapy. *Pediatr Rev.* 2019;40(5):219–228.

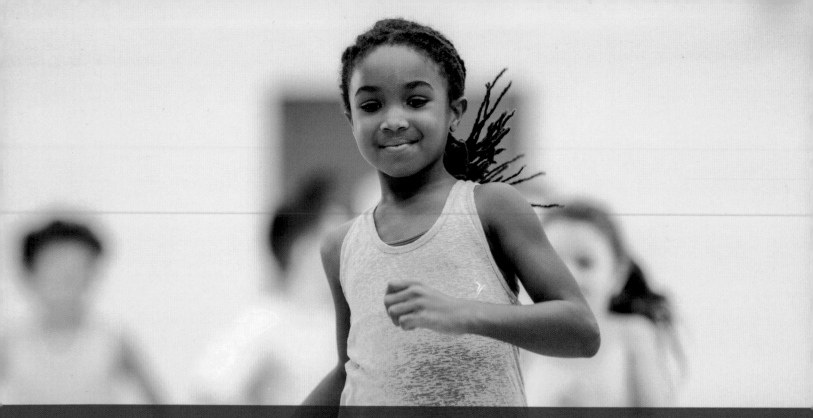

Effectively manage allergies, asthma, and pulmonary conditions with these AAP resources.

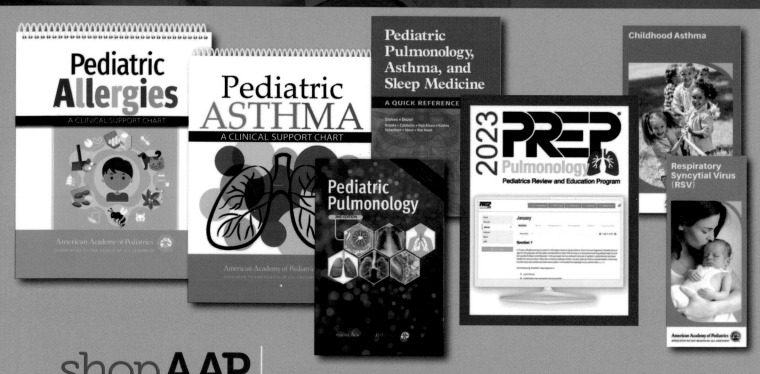